10-Day Bio

Metabolic Reset

10X SUPER HEALTH

PRESENTS

10-Day Bio Metabolic Reset

NATURAL WEIGHT LOSS, DISEASE PREVENTION AND CURES

www.10xsuperhealth.com

This publication contains the opinions and ideas of the author. It is intended for informational purposes only. The strategies in this program may not be suitable for every individual. Furthermore, it is provided with the understanding that neither the author nor the publisher are rendering any type of medical advice, and that the content is not intended to diagnose, treat, or cure any medical condition. If health or medical assistance is required, the services of a professional should be sought.

The author and publisher specifically disclaim any liability incurred from the use or application of the contents of this book. No particular results are guaranteed or warranted by using the information contained within.

Methods For Mastery, Inc.
PO Box 904
Wauna, WA 98395

First edition 2018

www.10xsuperhealth.com

This manual is a nonfictional work. Names and places have been changed to protect the privacy of all individuals. Any resulting resemblance to persons living or dead is entirely coincidental and unintentional. The events and situations are true.

Printed in the United States of America
ISBN 978-0-9905072-2-2

Dedicated to those who go the extra mile to figure out what is holding them back then crush it!

Warning - Consult a Physician

This should always be done before starting any diet or exercise program, including this one. If you are on any medications or other doctor prescribed treatments, it is even more essential. When followed, the 10-Day Bio Metabolic Reset has the potential to change your health condition dramatically. Things like taking prescriptions to lower your blood pressure could become unnecessary and taking them when you are healthy could actually put you at risk of too low blood pressure. That is just one example, but this type of regimen has led to the elimination of medications for multiple conditions. So, it is important to use caution and consult the necessary healthcare professionals before making any diet or lifestyle changes.

TABLE OF CONTENTS

INTRODUCTION

WHAT IS A BIO METABOLIC RESET

Over time, the Western Diet most of us have grown up on takes a nasty toll on our bodies. Unchecked, this can lead to all sorts of avoidable chronic diseases, weight gain, and even obesity. Your body has a natural ability to resist processed foods, chemicals, artificial substances, and other stresses put on it, but it has its limits.

These days, we live in a society filled primarily with an abundance of unhealthy foods our bodies were never designed to consume. Add to that the ever-increasing and pervasive use of pharmaceutical medications at a level we have never seen before and our bodies' natural defenses do not stand a chance. An abundance of unhealthy foods and pharmaceutical "remedies" for every ail, and our society is sicker than ever. This is a sign that we are exceeding the level of harmful substances our bodies can successfully defend against, which is resulting in an epidemic of predictable health decline and oftentimes premature death.

To alter the direction of these trends, we cannot continue on the same path and try to prescribe our way out of this. Therefore, the first step in preserving and restoring our health is to purge our system of the substances and toxic chemicals that are causing the harm. Then, we can flood our bodies with the vital nutrients that will help restore and reset its natural function and defense mechanisms. Regardless of what you have heard, your body is the only thing that can heal itself. No magic pills or potions necessary, all it needs are the natural ingredients on which it thrives, then it can do the rest.

So, a Bio Metabolic Reset is a strategic approach that works in harmony with your body to restore its biological and metabolic system functions naturally. The imbalance or compromised functions of these systems are what lead to illness and weight loss resistance. Your body is amazing. Given the proper environment, it can rebound from years of abuse and damage quicker than you might think.

Obviously, if you have 100 pounds to lose, this is not going to happen in 10 days. But, in 10 days, you can noticeably and dramatically change the direction of your health and rapidly accelerate the process of health restoration. The Bio Metabolic Resetting process will also help prepare your body for the journey back to good health. Trying to regain your health with a compromised body and a subtle approach can unnecessarily slow your progress, oftentimes leading to discouragement and failure from the resurfacing of old habits.

There is nothing subtle about the 10-Day Bio Metabolic Reset program. You will quickly be launched into weight loss of up to 10 pounds in just 10 days. And that is just the start. A good portion of that fat loss will be the unhealthy visceral fat that builds up around your organs. If you currently suffer from high blood pressure, you are likely to see a markedly beneficial move in the right direction. The unseen internal health improvements will be well under way, but you are also likely to notice many, if not all, of these more obvious improvements:

- Better Complexion
- Reduction in Body Size
- Increased Energy Level
- Improved Mental Clarity and Brain Function
- Improved Mood and Overall Wellbeing
- Less Body Aches

The list of benefits goes on and on, especially if you lead a 10X Super Health Lifestyle once you finish your 10-Day Reset. Those with high blood pressure and Type 2 Diabetes have a good chance they will substantially reduce their need for medication and possibly even get off it altogether.

WHY SHOULD YOU DO A RESET

Obesity, diabetes, heart disease, stroke, depression, and many other illnesses have become epidemics in the United States. We are the wealthiest and most medically advanced country in the world, but our health is in severe retreat. This is so out of control that, even with these advantages, life expectancy is expected to start decreasing. Below are just a few of the sobering statistics:

- **Adult Obesity Rate – 36.5%** (as of 2014 and increasing)
- **Children** 2-19 **Obesity Rate – 17%** (as of 2014 and increasing)
- **Americans with Diabetes – 30.3 million** or 9.4% of the population (2015 statistic)
- **Pre-Diabetic** Americans – **84.1 million** (2015 statistic)
- **Heart Disease Deaths – 610,000** It is the leading cause of death in America (2015 statistic)

- **High Blood Pressure – 32% of adults** only 54% have it under control (2015 statistic)

These statistics are alarming and unfortunately, due to the Western Diet, are still increasing. The worst part is that most could be greatly reduced or avoided all together, minimizing or eliminating the need for expensive and often ineffective medical treatment. I know that is a bold claim, and I am not intending to insult or disrespect the medical community in any way. Doctors and the medical establishment provide amazing and much-needed services that can help improve and even save people's lives. Just because they have that ability does not mean we should surrender our health in the hopes they can save us when our poor choices catch up with us. Due to the fact that doctors are highly trained in the medical field, many of us look to them for ways to maintain better health. This seems reasonable, until you consider that most receive very little, if any, training in the area of nutrition, which is the primary factor that determines your health.

Much scientific research has been done helping us understand the cause of these diseases, and we know how to prevent most of them, so why are alarm bells not going off and a major push to educate the American public about this being made? Currently, few in the medical community (it is a growing number but far from an acceptable level) and government are seriously looking to educate us and truly look out for our wellbeing, and there is good reason for that (the money). You have heard the saying an ounce of prevention is worth a pound of cure. Well, a million dollars of prevention could save a billion dollars in cure. If that is the case, do you want to be in the prevention business and work for the millions or focus on the billions available for the treatment? Sadly, some of these illnesses that are not prevented lead to death or become incurable, leading to a lifetime of treatment (can you hear big pharma and the medical mega corporations cheering?).

Enough about that. We all inherently know those things. So, what do we do about it? We take control and do what they do not want us to do, own our health, and that is exactly what I will show you how to do.

Associations

Before you go any further, take a few minutes to think through a few negative associations that you might have made in the past regarding your health habits that might not be serving you, then fill in the answers to the following questions. Keep in mind, your subconscious drives most of your habitual behavior without conscious thought. That fact has some good aspects to it but, unfortunately, some bad ones too.

The good is, you do not have to think about everything you do. The bad is, you do not think about everything you do. Your subconscious mind always intends to direct you in the best way possible, but if you have picked up bad habits in the past, your subconscious could be effortlessly driving you to repeat those actions to your detriment. So, take a few minutes now to work on your subconscious thinking with some conscious efforts.

Associations Exercise

List three negative associations you have made in the past about your diet and health that were not made by choice or with intention.

Some examples of negative associations might be: "I am just big boned" (this might have subconsciously given you permission to not watch your weight), or "I have to eat everything I put on my plate" (you are probably consuming more than you need and will be healthier if you do not), or maybe "My life is too hectic; I do not have time to cook at home" (in reality, there are easy to prepare healthy meals you can make at home that take no longer than going through the drive-thru. After you identify the negative association and how it has not been serving you, write down a new association to replace it.

My Associations

1. Association: _____

_____

_____

How has this negatively impacted your life?

_____

_____

_____

_____

What is a new, more empowering association with which you could replace this one?

_____

_____

_____

2. Association: _____

_____

_____

How has this negatively impacted your life?

_____

_____

_____

_____

What is a new more empowering association with which you could replace this one?

_____

_____

_____

3. Association: _____

_____

_____

How has this negatively impacted your life?

_____

_____

_____

_____

What is a new more empowering association with which you could replace this one?

_____

_____

_____

WHY SHOULD YOU DO A RESET

I hope you took this exercise seriously and put some real thought and effort into it. Some of the exercises in this program may not resonate with you or seem necessary, but consciously raising your awareness of your current self and the person you ultimately want to be can have a huge impact on your future behavior. Rest assured, if you take the actions outlined in this program, your time will not be wasted, and you will get the results you are after.

TWO MAJOR BONUSES FOR LONG-TERM HEALTH

Aside from the benefits previously mentioned, your 10-Day Reset also helps you conquer the hardest part of making two necessary changes required for long-term good health. These changes are breaking any sugar addiction and resetting your taste buds, so you actually like and desire the foods that lead to good health. These changes will not be fully complete or set in the 10-Days, but the hardest part will be done. Your old patterns (habits) will be interrupted and replaced with new beneficial ones. To finalize and make these changes permanent, continue implementing these healthier alternatives consistently for another 20 or more days. This will provide you the opportunity to establish some new lifelong 10X Super Health habits.

Your health is a result of your health habits. They are virtually effortless once set. I assume, if you are reading this, you have some less than ideal health habits. You perform these daily, as does everyone else, without conscious thought. They were likely created many years ago, without your intention or consent. Worse, they are likely based on some ill-advised and outdated health guidelines like, "Milk, it does the body good" or "Fat makes you fat." The great news is that, regardless of the source or how long you have had these habits, you can change them. Not in years, months or weeks, you can literally change them right now. To do this, here are two things you must do.

Breaking The Sugar Addiction

I do not know your true diet or condition, but a large percentage of people, especially Americans, have a sugar addiction. This addiction may not be obvious if you interpret sugar as the white powder or cubes. That sugar is one of the drugs that feed this addiction, but the sugar addiction I am actually taking about is better identified as a "blood sugar" addiction, otherwise known as blood glucose.

We have blamed the obvious added sugars, like the sugar in soda etc. for the increase in Type 2 Diabetes, but that is a dangerous conclusion. When we accept that conclusion, we allow ourselves to continue our sugar addiction; meanwhile, the epidemics of obesity, diabetes, and the other chronic illnesses of which 70%+/- are food related and avoidable through lifestyle changes continue. This gives big food manufactures a "license to kill" while they profit.

A blood sugar addiction is when we are hooked on the momentary high (good feelings) we get when we spike our blood sugar with foods or beverages. Unfortunately, it is not just sugar that causes these harmful, fat generating blood sugar spikes. It is actually a large percentage of what most people consume every day, things you would probably never expect, like orange juice, bread, pasta, oatmeal, cereal and the list goes on. In an attempt to be healthy, we drink diet soda (which is as bad or worse for you in the fat building process than non-diet versions) and watch how much sugar we add to our food. Watch all you like, but good luck avoiding it by just eliminating what you add. Food manufacturers have pretty much loaded everything with it to the perfect level, maximizing your blood sugar rush and peaking your cravings. They have got us hooked, so we keep coming back to our sugar addiction, destroying our health and our lives without pause.

During your 10-Day Bio Metabolic Reset, you will be going cold turkey without any of these blood sugar spiking drugs. This will get you through the toughest part of the detox process and accelerate your body's health recovery. This is, by far, the hardest and most challenging part of getting your health and weight under control, but this program is designed to make it as easy as possible. By the time you complete the 10-Day Reset, your strongest cravings will have subsided, and you will be experiencing the affects of better health. As I mentioned earlier, at this point, all you will need to do to complete this transition is steer clear of the addictive blood sugar spiking foods and beverages for an additional 20 days or more. I will cover the things to avoid in more detail in the following pages.

If you are truly committed to creating a lifestyle that naturally leads to good health, I recommend following your reset with the 10X Super Health Lifestyle program. The guidelines included in the "Life After Reset" chapter will give you everything you need to easily and consistently continue living a healthy lifestyle.

Resetting Your Taste Buds

The second bonus is major progress in the process of resetting your taste buds. This might sound a little funny. Who knew you could actually set these? Luckily, we not only set our taste preferences, but we also have the ability to reset them. Food manufacturers have known and used this fact for years to hijack our taste buds and steer us towards the foods they want to sell, cheap, easy and profitable. Yep, and they did this without regard for one key factor, our health. Let that be what it may, it is now our time to take back the reins and our health.

The 10-Day Reset will not change your taste buds all together; rather, it is the first phase of the process. This phase involves breaking your old taste preferences for unhealthy foods and freeing them to be reset to crave and appreciate the flavors that lead to great health. Why do most hate diets or resist the change to eating foods they know are much better for them? It is the thoughts of having to eat "healthy foods," when we are not fond of the flavor. That is totally understandable, but with a little effort, you can turn many of the healthy foods/flavors you may not currently like into those you will actually desire. The fact is, this is a must if you want to maintain good health for the long-term.

Our taste buds come with some preferences from the womb. They actually get pre-programmed from our mother's diet. Then they are developed further by the food selections we are exposed to in the early stages of life. If they are blood sugar spiking foods, we are setup for failure due to the addictive qualities of these unhealthy foods (some research has concluded they are more addictive than cocaine). As we get older, we develop preferences and start to consume more of the things we like. If we have developed a palette for blood sugar spiking foods, we will push away those that do not give us the high, possibly even throwing tantrums until our parents submit and give us another hit of the "good stuff."

This first step in transitioning your taste preferences is to neutralize your current taste cravings. If they are tuned for the addictive blood sugar spiking foods, this will be an uncomfortable process, but one you must go through to have a chance at a different outcome. Essentially, you are going to be getting weaned off a serious addiction and are likely going to experience some withdrawal symptoms. The fastest and most successful way to do this is cold turkey. Anything else will draw out the process, increasing the opening of time for failure. By the completion of your 10-Day Reset, you will have made it through the withdrawal period and made some major progress on breaking your old taste preferences.

One of the biggest reasons many of the largest and most commercially successful mainstream diet programs fail is because they sell you on the illusion that you can still eat the unhealthy foods you love. The only way that scenario works is if you are extremely disciplined and can live a lifetime of calorie restricted eating. So, can you? Even if you can, it is still a poor plan. Although you might lose weight and maintain the losses with this method, which can have some health benefits, you are likely just going to be eating smaller portions of unhealthy foods. Over the long term, this can lead to nutrient deficiencies and other chronic illnesses. Furthermore, most people cannot maintain a diet based on caloric restrictions. If you do crack and have not reset your palette (taste preferences), you will likely end up binge eating the same unhealthy foods to which you are accustomed. This is the root cause of the yo-yo dieting phenomenon.

Dangerous Food Manipulations

These days, many of the foods that make up the typical Western Diet have been manipulated for many reasons, but the outcome has been harmful and deceives our natural taste preferences. I am not talking about the extreme scientific versions, like GMOs, just simply plant cross-breeding and processing manipulations, many that seem harmless. Food was intended to be eaten in the most natural state possible. The Western Diet has changed the way we manufacture and consume our foods, leading to an epidemic of food related health issues. As these practices spread around the world, you can see the dramatic health impacts on the people in the communities adopting them.

We, as with all living organisms, naturally have built-in protection mechanisms designed to steer our choices and keep us safe. One of these is our taste palette. Foods that are inherently unhealthy or dangerous tend not to taste good, which is a sign we should not eat it. This is prevalent throughout nature. In fact, some plants give off toxins that are harmful to bugs to protect the plant. The bugs know this plant is deadly and will choose healthier options.

We are no different. This is especially true when it comes to things like grains. That is why many of the most common grains we eat today are highly modified. In their original forms, we would likely resist eating them; their taste is less than desirable. Wheat in its natural whole grain form is not very tasty to most. This should be our sign to stay away and not eat it. But, due to its cheap, easy to produce, and desirable shelf-life attributes, they have found ways to modify and process it in ways that appeal to our palettes. This modification process (in the case of wheat, refining, among other things) makes the flavor more tolerable and, to some, even appealing. So now, we are open to eating foods that have been made unhealthy. Worse yet, due to the refining process, it has actually been made even unhealthier by manipulating it into an extremely efficient blood sugar spiking and addictive food.

This is just one example but a prevalent one that affects the health of most. We will be going more in-depth on these topics later, but the point is that you understand your taste preferences are under your control, and you can change them to serve you. Done properly, these changes can help you acquire taste preferences for foods that are natural and provide real health benefits. This will help you stay on the path to a healthy lifestyle, one that includes the ability to maintain a healthy weight more easily.

10-DAY BIO METABOLIC RESET

LIFESTYLE MATTERS

When it comes to health, most people think of diet and exercise as being what counts. Obviously, those are the primary components, but successfully achieving and maintaining good health can benefit greatly from looking beyond the obvious factors. Some of these lifestyle elements have the potential to undermine large portions of any diet and exercise improvements you make, so they are well-worth understanding and paying attention to.

The 10X Super Health philosophy is based on living a lifestyle that supports good health naturally. We all know diets do not work long term, and it makes sense, because they are just an event. These events are meant to create change, and many do, but upon completion, we tend to fall back into the environment and habits that create the unhealthy lifestyle in the first place.

To be clear, the 10-Day Bio Metabolic Reset is a short-term event. It is not intended or suitable for long-term use. The purpose of this program is to break old habits quickly, detoxify and cleanse your body, help you break any sugar addiction, and reset your taste buds, freeing you of preferences for unhealthy and processed foods.

I have included a Life After Reset Guide within this book to help you transition into a healthy lifestyle suitable for long-term use. Fortunately, many aspects of this program are not only compatible but beneficial parts of that lifestyle. When used long term, they will help you maintain good health and your ideal body weight, without substantial effort or constant dieting.

Note: *This is not a book of science. It is a book based on science. What that means is, some of the subject matters could go very deep scientifically, which would make this book unnecessarily long. That is not the goal; rather, it has been designed to give you actionable steps you can take to get the results, while providing a general understanding of the supporting science behind them.*

INTERMITTENT FASTING

Intermittent fasting is very popular these days and for good reason. There are many great benefits that can come from practicing it. Numerous studies have been done verifying these facts, and due to the positive results, it is catching on. Some of these benefits are:

- Weight Loss
- Increased Energy
- Increased Memory and Better Brain Health
- Reduces Insulin Resistance
- Heart Health
- Anti-Aging Attributes

And those are just some of the benefits. I am not going to go deep into each of these benefits, as the value for this program is the sum of the whole. We are looking to detox your system and reboot it, so all these elements are beneficial, supportive, and in alignment with the objective.

There are many different methods of intermittent fasting, some lasting for hours, others for days. Each have their own merits and purpose, but for this program, we will just look to extend the daily fast we all currently do each night. Our goal is 16 hours of fasting per day. The exact timing is not important, only that the hours be consecutive.

Our bodies are designed to go through feasts and famine, so during feasts it stores energy to be used during times of famine. This energy is primarily stored as fat, and fat is filled with toxins, so our goal is to purge as much fat and toxins from our bodies as possible. Your body responding to a famine, even if it is only for 16 hours, will be of great help in achieving that goal.

I recommend starting your fast around dark or shortly thereafter, working with your circadian rhythm to maximize the results. You can experiment with what timing works best for you; just try to go for 16 hours straight once you begin your fast. The first few days will be the most challenging, but soon your body will adapt to this new routine.

You might be thinking there is no way I can do this. 16 hours with no food? Do not stress. There are ways to make this, not only doable, but also tolerable. Not only will it be easier than you think, the way you will feel after doing it for 10 days will make it well worth it.

A lot of people think of a fast as starving, but you do not have to go hungry for a fast to be effective. The goal is to postpone activating your digestive system during your fast. You can do this by avoiding carbs, protein, and sugars. My secret to extending a fast to 16 hours successfully is by having a cup of 10X Fasting Tea in the morning when I start to feel hungry. This will temporarily eliminate any hunger pangs and give you more time before you need to break your fast.

10X Fasting Tea

So, what is 10X Fasting Tea? It is a recipe of black tea, MCT oil, and coconut oil that I created to make fasting more comfortable while providing additional benefits. The oils not only help you avoid feeling hungry, but this recipe will give you energy, ignite your brain function, and help you enter a mild state of ketosis. During ketosis, your body converts fat into ketones and burns them as its main source of energy. Since our goal is to burn fat and eliminate toxins, this is of great benefit.

I have included the recipe in the Reset Recipes section of this book, but essentially, you will brew some black tea, add your MCT and coconut oil, then infuse it by mixing it in a bullet or other high-speed blending device.

CIRCADIAN RHYTHM

We all have something called a circadian rhythm, which affects us in some pretty dramatic ways, especially when it comes to weight loss or more typically weight gain. This rhythm runs in constant 24-hour cycles and helps key functions of our bodies effortlessly adjust and keep us in harmony. Some of these adjustments help us sleep when it make sense (it is dark out), while others help synchronize our digestion to be fired up when we are likely to be eating (it is light out).

So why does it matter, and how does this affect our weight loss/gain? This system was designed to support us in our natural environment, long before the invention of commercial food manufacturing process, grocery stores, and 24-hour light available at the flip of a switch. This affects our ability and the likelihood we will be eating at times that are out of synchronization with the way our bodies are optimized to eat and process food. If we work in harmony with the design of our bodies, we will be less prone to weight gain. We can also leverage this natural occurrence to help aid in the process of weight loss when necessary. Light-based fasting and time-based eating are key strategies for successfully leveraging the full power of the 10X Super Health Lifestyle.

Circadian Based Intermittent Fasting

As mentioned before, there are many variations of intermittent fasting. These tactics are typically based on timeframes like fasting 10-12 hours a day or for an entire day at certain intervals. Those all would likely be of some benefit, but when we look at the natural laws that are the foundation for our circadian rhythm functions, I believe light-based fasting is the best method for determining when and how long the ideal fast should be. That being said, while doing your 10-Day Reset, I advise using the principles of the Light Based Fasting method while stretching the length to 16 hours.

Light Based Fasting – Our biological rhythm supports a philosophy of eating when it is naturally light out, when we could see to hunt, prepare, and eat our food. Therefore, working off a rule of avoiding eating when it is dark outside works in harmony with our bodies' natural process. This is supported by the second key element necessary for leveraging the circadian rhythm.

Time-Based Eating

Our bodies' insulin response to food is dramatically different based on what time of day it is. This is relevant because insulin is responsible for turning an overabundance of glucose (a simple sugar in your blood) into fat for use at a later time.

We tend to produce a much larger insulin response when eating in the evening compared to only a small response in the morning. So, why is there a difference in insulin production based on the time of day? This is likely because our body functions are based on the assumption that we have not been eating all night. Therefore, we are likely low in blood sugar and will need and are able to use what is provided in a breakfast meal. On the other hand, the response to eating in the evening would be based on the assumption that you will likely be resting or sleeping soon. Based on that, there will not be a high demand for energy, so your body is designed to capture and store that abundance of energy (as fat) for later use.

The conflict in design and use comes down to the fact that your body is designed to store abundances of energy for a future time of famine, which in the past was frequent. These days, we have plenty of food available 24/7, so no famines in sight. Therefore, we just keep packing on layer upon layer of fat as we overconsume. Even worse, we often do it at the ideal times for fat creation (dinner). So, what can we do differently to avoid packing on this unwanted fat?

Eat Major Meals Early – Forget the traditional Western eating pattern, which includes a large meal for dinner and is oftentimes followed with a sweet desert. That is a huge mistake! Not only will your system produce a large amount of insulin that will immediately store a good portion of your meal as fat, but it is perfectly primed to spike your insulin and turn any sugar or carbs from desert into fat. The best approach is to consume the largest portion of your food/calories in the AM and early afternoon. If you do eat in the evening, try to focus on smaller portions of low carb and low sugar foods. High carb and high sugar foods paired with the already large insulin response will promote even more fat creation.

Benefits

By providing your body with the nutrients and calories it needs at the times it is optimally designed to use them, you will be able to put more of them to work as energy and store less as fat. These eating times and the fast when it is dark method may seem like a challenge, and no doubt, it will be initially. Luckily, as you develop and spend more time living a 10X Super Health Lifestyle, these things will become easier and more natural. Eventually, these beneficial changes can become your habitual actions that require no extra effort or intention.

The types and abundance of foods these days make weight and health management a challenge. Working to maximize the benefits of some or all of these lifestyle strategies can help give you the upper hand. No single food or strategy can work alone. It takes the combination of consistent small, healthy choices to get and maintain optimum health. Build habits around these choices, and good health will be the effortless byproduct.

SLEEPING OFF THE POUNDS

We have all heard and know we need to get enough sleep each night, 7 to 9 hours for most people. But if you are struggling to maintain or lose weight, this is even more critical advice for you to heed. Not getting enough sleep can dramatically reduce our ability to lose or keep weight off. According to some studies, your ability to lose or avoid gaining weight can be reduced by over 50% compared to someone who gets adequate sleep.

These days, getting enough sleep is not as easy as it once was. With high levels of stress, overbooked schedules, and more to get done than the hours in the day allow, even if you do have the time required, many people have trouble getting to sleep and or achieving the most beneficial deep sleep. If this is you, I do not recommend taking pills to assist in obtaining more sleep. Pharmaceuticals as sleep aids, as well as for just about anything else, tend to have a plethora of negative side effects. Here are a few drug-free strategies that might be helpful in increasing the amount and quality of sleep you get.

Adequate Time – Arrange your schedule and allot yourself adequate time to get a minimum of at least 7 hours of sleep each night. Do not hop into bed 7 hours before your alarm is set to go off and expect to get 7 hours of sleep. I recommend being in bed with at least the amount of desired sleep time plus one hour before your alarm goes off. This will give you some buffer time to fall asleep, as well as cover sleep lost from getting up to use the restroom or other sleep interruptions.

Screen Time – Avoid electronic screen time for two hours prior to going to sleep. I know this can be hard. Since the invention of our virtual lives on Facebook, Smart Phones, and the ability to binge watch Netflix, it is easier and more tempting than ever. Going out of your way to accomplish this is worth it, especially if you are trying to lose some weight or want to bring your sharpest mind to a task.

Night Shades – Use blackout night shades to eliminate changes in light that can trigger your circadian rhythm's wakeup response. If you have trouble getting sound sleep and have never tried this, give it a shot. Just be sure to set a good alarm, because you may find yourself sleeping a couple hours longer than you anticipate.

Meditation – This may sound a little to esoteric for some, but doing a little self-directed meditation or listening to a guided meditation designed as a sleep aid can work wonders. These methods are intended to get us out of our head and calm the mind, which allows for an easy transition into sleep. This does not have to be time consuming. 10-15 minutes should be adequate.

Other Tricks – Here are a few more simple strategies that are known to assist in better sleep.

- Maintain a consistent sleep schedule
- Exercise during the day
- Make sure your room is cool
- Avoid caffeine, alcohol, eating (especially carbs and sugars) or drinking other beverages within a few hours of bedtime

Do not unnecessarily undermine your efforts. Stepping up, putting in the effort, and taking the steps necessary to lose weight and gain better health is commendable. You deserve to achieve the best results. Whether it is prioritizing more time or eliminating or adding something new to your sleep plan, make sure adequate sleep is part of your healthy lifestyle.

Interesting Fact - *In the "Whitehall II Study," British researchers discovered that getting less than 5 hours of sleep each night doubles the risk of death from cardiovascular disease. Worse yet, according to the CDC, cardiovascular disease is the #1 cause of death in the United States.*

STRESS VS HEALTH

Stress is a bad thing. We have all heard the reports and read the stories, and frankly, it just does not feel good. It turns out, it not only feels bad, but it shortens our lives and contributes to weight gain. There are two primary ways that high levels of stress can limit attempts to lose weight or, worse yet, actually cause us to gain weight.

Cortisol – When you are stressed, your body creates the hormone cortisol, which can lead to weight gain. This is due to the fact that it increases insulin production (the fat builder), while at the same time lowers your blood sugar, which leads to increased cravings for sweet foods. This is the perfect recipe for violating any good intentions and emotionally eating foods that will rapidly be turned into fat.

Fight or Flight Response – Second, our innate response of "fight or flight" is triggered during stressful times. This can often lead to overeating in an attempt to comfort our heightened emotions and help us relax. These two stress related conditions make reducing or eliminating stress a requirement for good health.

Reducing Stress

With high cortisol production and the fight or flight response working against us, we obviously want to do whatever we can to help reduce or eliminate our stresses. Success in this area is not always easy, but here are a few things you might want to try.

Exercise – Not only is this beneficial to our health and weight loss goals, but it is also known as being one of the most effective ways to reduce stress. Exercising is known for reducing our level of harmful stress hormones and can have therapeutic mental benefits, leading to an improved mood and state of wellbeing.

Connections – Spending time with your deepest connections, whether human, pets, hobbies, or other interests, can help put your mind at ease and reduce stress levels. Prioritizing and increasing the amount of time spent with these connections can be a beneficial part of meeting any stress reduction goals.

Minimize Procrastination – Procrastination is easy to do, especially when you are stressed.

Unfortunately, this tends to contribute to even higher levels of stress. So, try to make it a priority to push yourself to do those things you might be putting off.

Laugh – It might take something really funny to break us out of a stressed state, but laughter, if you can achieve it, might just be the cure you are looking for. It is extremely hard. Actually, it is next to impossible to be stressed out when you are laughing. Whether you get these laughs from a funny movie or some other source does not really matter. Even a short interruption to a stressful state can have long-term benefits.

Stress Reduction Plan

If stress is an issue, make lightening your stress load a short-term goal. Identify the areas and stresses in your life and create an action plan to help reduce or eliminate any you might have. Take a minute to write down a few things that cause you stress and some steps you can take to help minimize or eliminate them.

Stress: _____

_____

Stress Elimination Plan: _____

_____

_____

_____

_____

Stress: _____

_____

Stress Elimination Plan: _____

_____

_____

_____

_____

Stress: _____

_____

Stress Elimination Plan: _____

_____

_____

_____

_____

ACTIVITY PLAN

Increase Activity Level – While performing a 10-Day Bio Metabolic Reset, high levels of exercise are not required. That being said, your results will be enhanced by using your muscles and moving more.

Weight loss is a result of this program, not the focus. The focus is cleaning your body of fat and toxins while quickly moving you into a better state of health. If you live a sedentary or minimally active lifestyle, adding at least 10% more activity of any type will be a major benefit towards improving your overall state of health. Below are 3 simple ways to add more activity to your lifestyle without taking any additional time out of your day.

1. **Act Immediately** – When you think about wanting or doing something that is not within your reach, go get it. Do not wait until it is convenient or decide to go without. This will make you more effective and add movement to your lifestyle. Standing up, walking across the

room and back, actually has great health benefits. Every extra time you do this will help, so try to do it more often.

2. **Hustle** – Put a little more kick in your step. When walking or doing something, just do it a little faster or with a little higher rate of intensity. You burn approximately twice as many calories per minute running a mile as you do walking one. That makes sense. You are exercising more rigorously, so of course, you will burn more in the same time. Here is the thing; take time out of the equation, and you will still burn about 25% more energy covering one mile running as you do walking it. So, increasing your intensity of movement can increase your caloric burn for the same task. Not to mention, if you are moving or doing things faster, you are actually improving your health while getting more done in the same or even less time.

3. **Strategically Increase Activity Requirement** – This can include simple things, like taking the stairs, parking further out in the parking lot, walking the dog, doing some yard work, cleaning the house etc. An add is an add, and many can be productive, giving you more than just health benefits and an increase in caloric burn.

SUCCESS SUPPORT

For many, this may not be the first program they have
tried; in fact, it may only be one of many. This is not
surprising, as change can be hard, and because of
this, I recommend building some support resources
to help ensure your success. Support can come in
many forms, and the more types you use, the better
your chances of overcoming the challenges that tend
to lead to failure.

Support Plan

Below are a few key areas you should consider
focusing some attention on and proactively create a
support action plan.

Environment – This is one of the most controllable
and most powerful success tools there is. Help
yourself avoid temptations by making adjustments to
your environment in advance, thereby limiting your
exposure to them. Things like removing snacks you
typically enjoy from your cabinets and avoiding

meetings at Starbucks when you know you can not resist the temptations are good ideas. Aside from avoiding temptations, you can intentionally put yourself in positive environments that support good health. This might include things like using a local walking path where other people are out getting exercise. Identify and make a plan to address some temptations you need to eliminate and possible supportive environments where you might benefit from spending more time.

People – There have been studies regarding the effects of the top few people we hang around with rubbing off on us. This happens in both good and bad ways. This is due to the fact that they support and promote their good and/or bad habits, which creates an unseen energy that tends to influence our choices and is hard to resist. I am not suggesting you disassociate from those you know and love. Although limiting the time you spend around anyone that might be a less than supportive association for some period of time could be to your advantage.

It is also a good idea to increase the time spent around those that you feel can play supportive roles in this endeavor, maybe even get them to join you for this challenge. Let those in your inner circle know exactly what you are doing and what your goals are. Ask them directly for their support and tell them what they can do to help you succeed. The process of making this clear and getting it out in the open in advance will not be an act in vain. This will align your support team. Not only will it help align them with your mission, but this direct request will make them feel more accountable for their actions, improving the odds that they will maintain a supportive role.

Immersion – If you really want to master your health, it needs to be your focus. Until you have successfully adopted the new actions and habits you desire, spending your free energy and time learning about and practicing the skills required will help keep you on track. This might come in the form of reading and researching, taking a course or program, or anything else that immerses you in something associated with your objective. It takes approximately 30 days for most people to replace and develop a new habit that sticks. So it is a good idea to remain consistent and immersed for at least that long.

Support Action Plan

Use the following space to document any thoughts or ideas you have that might help you create a strong supportive environment. Just the simple act of getting clear and writing out your thoughts and plans increases the chances that you will remember and follow through with enacting them.

Support Action Plan

_____

_____

_____

_____

_____

_____

_____

_____

_____

_____

_____

_____

_____

_____

_____

GETTING STARTED

You do not need much to get started on this program, but you will need a few things before you get going. Obviously, you are going to need some food, but you will also need a few tools and accessories. The following list includes the things you need and those you might want just to make things a little easier or to help you connect to the process. I have noted the items that are essential, along with my recommended solution. For a complete guide and the most up to date recommendations list, go to:

www.10xsuperhealth.com/essentials/

Do not get hung up on the optional items. They are great to have, but the most important thing is to get started.

Tools and Accessories

Extractor (required) – This is the key piece of equipment you will need and be using daily. As with anything, there are numerous options on the market. Here are my top recommendations.

- **NutriBullet** (600 Watts) – This is the minimum piece of equipment I would recommend, but it is not ideal.
- **NutriBullet Pro** (900 Watts) – This is the mid-range model and my favorite when it comes to performance. I use this model.
- **NutriBullet RX** (1200 Watts) – This model works better for families or when mixing multiple beverages at once, I also use this model. Between the two, I prefer using the Pro model unless I am mixing large drinks and need the extra capacity, but either will get the job done.

Note: *A blender is not adequate to extract the nutrients from the ingredients. A typical household blender may seem suitable, but I highly recommend you use an actual extractor during the Bio Reset. These machines have more power and higher speeds, which allow them to extract nutrients from seeds and other ingredients. These are also very useful long term as a part of your 10X Super Health Lifestyle.*

Body Weight Scale (required – recommend digital) – You will be weighing yourself daily and want an accurate and easy to use scale.

Shaker Bottle (optional) – You need something to drink your smoothie out of. These work great because some beverages tend to separate as they sit. These also work great for storing/refrigerating smoothies for later, as you can remix by just giving the container a little shake. A glass is also a perfectly adequate solution.

Water Bottle (optional) – I highly recommend getting in the habit of using a re-usable water bottle. This is handy for multiple reasons. One, you can take it with you and always have it; two, you can use it to measure and keep track of how much fluid you are taking in each day. Not to mention, it is also much more environmentally friendly when compared to the throwaway water bottles.

Compost Bin (optional) – This was a must for me, since I have a garden. It makes handling the abundance of compostable food scraps easy to deal with, while minimizing odor.

Food Scale (optional) – I found this very handy when I got started. Food nutrition is oftentimes given in grams per serving, and I frankly did not know how to guess how much a gram is. I have tried to be very descriptive with the ingredients, so you do not necessarily need a scale, but for the price, they are handy when you do.

Storage Containers (optional) – You may have something that will work for this purpose. If not, I have found Snapware's BPA free, square grip canisters to be a convenient and easy to use solution.

Other Things (required) – These are pretty typical, so you probably have them floating around your kitchen.

1. Cutting Board
2. Knives
3. Measuring Spoons and Cups
4. Assorted Storage Containers

Food

I have included a few specific ingredient lists to help you shop and track your consumption. These are custom-tailored to your ideal target weight and can be found in the 10-Day Program section.

Why These Ingredients

Each ingredient used in this reset has been specifically chosen to deliver specific health benefits and help you achieve the overall goal. As they are all great ingredients, many have similar benefits as well as their own unique nutritional aspects; the following brief descriptions are the primary benefits that warrant their inclusion.

Apples

Apples contain many nutrients, vitamins, and minerals and are a good source of antioxidants and soluble fiber. These features aid in digestion, help prevent inflammation, support good gut bacteria, lower bad cholesterol, and so much more. Among other things, this helps lower the risks of heart disease, stroke, and cancer.

Sauerkraut

This is a powerful resource when it comes to restoring good gut flora and reducing bad bacteria. It also boosts your immune system, improves digestion, helps reduce stress, contributes to stronger bones and overall heart health. Sauerkraut's flavor is not for everyone, but the benefits are well-worth getting over any flavor objections. Be sure it is the raw unpasteurized type that will be found in the refrigerated section of your grocery store. You also want to choose the one with the least amount of ingredients (ideally, just sauerkraut and salt).

Watermelon

Watermelon is loaded with antioxidants, vitamins, and amino acids. It contains toxin fighting nutrients that aid your liver in the detoxification process. It is also a great hydration source that helps lower cholesterol, boosts immunity, and may help fight cancer.

Grapefruit

Grapefruit supports weight loss by boosting your metabolism, is high in fiber, aids in lowering cholesterol and blood pressure. It is also shown to support skin health and appearance, boost your immunity, and fight cancer.

Lemon

Lemons are loaded with nutrients and vitamins that are known to aid in digestion, weight loss, and heart health. Like grapefruit, it supports skin health, helps fight cancer, and increases iron absorption.

Frozen Berry Mix

Berries are a super food loaded with inflammation fighting antioxidants, high in fiber, and may help inhibit the development of some cancers. It has also been shown to boost brain and heart health.

Cucumber

Cucumbers are a low calorie, hydrating food with disease fighting properties. They are high in antioxidants and have been shown to have anti-cancer and anti-inflammatory qualities. They also aid in the detoxification process, alkalize blood, support strong bones and heart health.

Celery

Celery lowers inflammation, helps lower blood pressure, can reduce bad cholesterol, and is a great liver cleansing food. As well, it boosts digestion and can reduce bloating.

Leafy Greens (spinach or kale)

These are excellent sources of vitamins, minerals, antioxidants, and a powerful anti-inflammatory food. They contain insoluble fiber, which aids in digestion, have been shown to aid in detoxification, help prevent heart disease and fight cancer.

Broccoli

Packed with vitamins, nutrients, and antioxidants, broccoli is great for helping lower inflammation and may protect against cancer. It is beneficial for heart health, blood sugar control, supports good digestion, strong bones and healthy gut bacteria.

Ginger

Ginger promotes gut health, fights fungal infections, is anti-inflammatory, is an antimicrobial, has been shown to have anti-cancer benefits, lowers cholesterol, and supports good liver health.

Beets

Beets are high in nutrients and antioxidants while being low in calories. They are known for supporting good athletic performance, weight loss, aid in detoxification, help regulate blood pressure, improve digestion, and have anti-cancer properties.

Almonds

Almonds are loaded with healthy fats and fiber that can aid in weight loss. They promote brain health, blood sugar control, heart health, can help fight cancer and inflammation, while increasing nutrient absorption and digestion. They also support hair and skin health.

Flaxseeds

Flaxseeds are high in fiber and omega-3 fatty acids, while being low in carbs. They are also high in antioxidants, support lower cholesterol, good digestion, as well as skin and hair health.

Chia Seeds

Chia seeds are loaded with nutrients and anti-oxidants. They are also high in fiber, protein, and omega-3 fatty acids. Almost all their carbs are from the fiber. They are beneficial supporters of good heart health, boost energy, build strong bones, fight cancer growth, and aid in the detoxification process.

Coconut Water

Coconut water is low in calories, high in potassium, is a good source of calcium, magnesium, and amino acids. Aids in detoxification, electrolyte replacement, and lowering cholesterol.

MCT Oil

Contains medium chain triglyceride fats. MCT Oil promotes weight loss, heart health, digestion, nutrient absorption, supports your good gut bacteria, provides a good source of immediately usable energy, and helps you feel full. It also has antiviral, antifungal, and antibacterial properties.

Coconut Oil

Also contains medium chain triglyceride fats that help boost fat burning while providing your body and mind with a good source of energy. Coconut oil has saturated fats that promote good heart health, can help raise the good HDL cholesterol in your blood, while reducing hunger, which can help you eat less. It can also help reduce inflammation, as well as aid in the prevention and treatment of cancer.

Cinnamon

Cinnamon helps balance blood sugar, improve weight loss, is a powerful antioxidant, anti-inflammatory, and helps protect against cardiovascular disease. It also fights infections, viruses, and may help lower the risk of some cancers.

Protein Powder

Having adequate amounts of protein helps protect your lean muscle mass when on low or super low calorie diets. It also takes double the calories to metabolize protein, which is known as the thermic effect. Protein based foods also tend to be more satisfying, helping reduce your cravings to eat more.

Vitamin B-12

Vitamin B-12 is an essential nutrient that helps boost energy, brain function, and the creation of red blood cells. It also supports heart, nervous system, and memory health.

Liver Rescue Supplement

The herbs in this supplement help support your liver detoxification process.

Colon Cleanse

Helps with bloating, removing harmful toxins, improved digestion, regularity, and the restoration of good bacteria in the colon.

Probiotic Supplement

Helps replenish the beneficial gut bacteria required for proper digestion and a strong immune system. Helps support vitamin production and an improved metabolism.

Green Tea

Green tea is loaded with polyphenols that help reduce inflammation and catechin, which is an antioxidant known for improving blood flow, lowering cholesterol, and helping with heart related issues, like high blood pressure and congestive heart failure. Green tea is also known to promote weight loss and lower the risks of cancer.

Black Tea

Black tea is high in antioxidants, increases energy, and has been shown to improve heart health while lowering the risk of stroke.

Apple Cider Vinegar

This is a beneficial contributor to the detoxification and good gut bacteria restoration process. It can also help lower cholesterol, aid in weight loss, lower blood pressure, and improve skin health. Your apple cider vinegar should be the raw type with the mother included (this makes it look murky, which is exactly what you want).

Water

Drinking adequate amounts of water can boost metabolism, increase energy levels, improve brain function, and help your body flush toxins.

Universal Program Guidelines

The following is an outline of the things you will be doing for each of the next 10 days to complete your Bio Metabolic Reset successfully. Although it is not critical to complete these in a specific fashion, it can be beneficial, so I have included an Example Daily Reset Strategy that you may wish to follow.

Measure – First thing each morning, eliminate (use the bathroom) and then hop on the scale and weigh yourself. Record this information on the Results Log located in the back of this book. For accurate results, wear the same clothes, if any, each time you weight yourself.

10X Fasting Tea – Each morning when you begin to feel hunger pangs, consume your fasting tea. Try to avoid anything else until you have successfully achieved a 16 hour fast since your last meal. If you can not make it the full 16 hours, go for as long as you possibly can and try to stretch a little longer each day until you reach the full term.

Breaking Fast, Morning Re-Hydration – Before consuming anything else, drink a glass of warm Apple Cider Vinegar Detoxer (program essential).

Must Do's – Due to your diet being 100% plant based during this 10-Day Bio Metabolic Reset, you need to make sure that each day you supplement the things that will not be adequately provided. The supplements to compensate adequately are listed below. Just make sure, if you skip anything, it is not one of these.

1. **Vitamin B12** – Any quality supplement will do, just be sure it has at least 25mcg of vitamin B12. Higher levels are ok as long as you do not exceed recommended dosage.
2. **Flaxseed** – Flaxseed is a good source of Omega-3 fatty acids (these are essential). Consume a minimum of 2 tablespoons a day of ground flaxseed. Your body cannot get the nutrients from flaxseed without the seed being broken open, so get ground flax or grind/extract it before you consume it (be sure to refrigerate after grinding to retain the beneficial nutrients).

Activating Your Digestion – Eating some crunchy ingredients traditionally (by chewing) helps activate your digestive acids and enzymes. So snacking on celery, almonds or other whole ingredients is a good thing.

Consume All Ingredients – Consume all the remaining ingredients on your eating plan, either as outlined or per your own custom strategy.

Water – Any water used for your morning re-hydration/Apple Cider Vinegar Detoxer, or for tea counts towards your daily minimum. Consume the balance throughout the day.

Supplements

Here is a brief overview of the supplements you should use during the program. Not all of these are required, but all are recommended for the best results.

Required: B12 – As mentioned, there are no sources of B12 in a plant-based diet, so you should use a supplement to obtain it. Any good B12 supplement will do, as long as it has at least 25mcg and is taken daily.

Required: Protein Powder – This should be plant-based (I recommend one with pea as the primary protein containing ingredient. Do not worry, it does not taste like peas). Do not use whey, soy, or other animal-based products. Look for one that is also a good source of iron; somewhere between 20-40% per serving is ideal. These will typically come in vanilla, chocolate or other flavors. Choose the one you prefer.

Liver Detox/Cleanse – Choose a high-quality liver detox and cleanse supplement that has at least 500 mg of Milk Thistle seed extract and 200 mg of Dandelion Root extract.

Colon Cleanse – Look for a blend that contains at least the following ingredients, Senna Leaves, Psyllium Husks, Cascara Sagrada Bark. As these are typically propriety blends, they will also likely contain many other ingredients, which is ok.

Pro-Biotic – Once again, choose a high-quality non-GMO version that has a high quantity of organisms. Around 40 billion is ideal.

For a complete list of supplements, their purposes and benefits, as well as links to the exact products I recommend, visit:

www.10xsuperhealth.com/supplements/

Excluded Detrimentals

Do not consume any of the items on the list below during your reset. I know some of these are addictions and may be hard to eliminate for even a short time, but if you truly want or need to regain your health, it is important that you at least eliminate these while doing the 10-Day Reset.

Avoid These Things

Soda	Eating Out
Juices (artificial or real)	Alcohol
Sports Drinks	Smoking Tabaco
Coffee Shop Beverages	Artificial Sweeteners

Tips and Warnings

Coffee – If you are a coffee drinker, abruptly giving this up during this period may lead to uncomfortable headaches or other withdrawal symptoms. Drinking coffee during your 10-Day Reset is not recommended but will only modestly affect your overall results. That being said, if you must have it, drink it without added sugar, artificial sweeteners, flavoring additives, dairy, or other creamers. Stevia can be used for sweetening or flavor enhancement.

Hunger Pangs – This program has been specifically designed to optimize your bio metabolic resetting process and lose weight. Due to this fact, there may be times during the first few days when you feel discomfort from hunger pangs. Depending on your past eating habits, this may be more or less extreme. Should the discomfort become more than you can handle, be prepared with the best remedies possible. Any added food or snacks will negatively affect your results and therefore are not recommended. If you do breakdown, minimize the impact by using more of the 10-Day Reset ingredients or choosing from the following list. Only consume the minimum amount you need to kill your hunger pangs.

1. **Nuts** – Raw unsalted Almonds or Walnuts. These are filled with healthy fats that will help satiate you. They also have some crunch that you might be missing.
2. **Avocado** – Filled with healthy fats that satiate.
3. **Almond Butter** – Once again, filled with healthy fats that satiate (must be real and organic with only two ingredients, the nuts and salt). Put this on some of your celery for added crunch factor.

My assumption is, if you are doing this, you desire obtaining noticeable results quickly. If that is true, I advise you to tough it out for the duration without cheats. The discipline and willpower required to follow through on big life changes, especially weight loss, can be hard to come by. The longer it drags on to get the results, the more likely we are to give up and fall back into our old habits. Fast and dramatic progress can be encouraging and help us stick it out through the hard times, so just go for it!

Constipation – For some people, a major diet change, especially if their system is compromised and in need, can lead to constipation. Due to the fact that this is a detox and you will be processing a lot of toxins, we want to make sure we keep you moving regularly. While on this program, you should have regular daily bowel movements. If this is not true for you, a few things you might want to try are:

- The Supplement Mag07
- An Herbal Tea with Senna

Pharmaceutical based laxatives are not recommended and should be considered a last resort. The overuse of pharmaceutical medications is one of the major contributors to compromised health, compromised organ functions, and the need to detox in the first place.

Weight Fluctuation – Do not expect your weight to go down every day. You should expect some fluctuations. This is normal and should not be a reason for concern. There are many reasons for this, but all you should worry about is that the predominate long-term trend is down.

Expect Some Discomfort – It is best to expect and plan for some discomfort. This is definitely a major life change that will get rapid results, so it is only reasonable to expect some hardships. These symptoms, if incurred, are transitional and will be short-lived. Do not try this if you will be traveling or on vacation. Also, try to do it when you will be able to manage a lower stress level. Keeping busy and minimizing environments that provide temptations for unhealthy habits of the past will help make things more bearable. Here are a few other temporary discomforts you may incur:

- Headache
- Fatigue
- Nausea
- Irritability
- Frequent urination
- Sleep disruption
- Cravings

Believe it or not, experiencing any of these is actually a positive sign. They are telling you that this was very necessary and that it is working. Rest assured, with a little willpower, you will get through this brief period just fine.

Freezing – You can prepare, cut, portion, individually bag, and freeze some of your fruits and vegetables. This is especially handy if you will be using these ingredients in smoothies, as it will help chill your beverage. For suitable ingredients, freezing will also help extend their shelf-life.

Bulk Preparation – You can prepare all your daily smoothies at the same time for convenience. This will greatly reduce your cleaning and daily interruption. Just be sure to refrigerate them in a sealed container with the least amount of air space possible to retain the maximum nutritional value.

Shelf Life Expectations – Your smoothies can be made in advance as long as you refrigerate them immediately and store them in sealed containers with minimal air space. Refrigerated, they can last a couple of days, but to maximize their nutritional benefits, I recommend consuming them within 24+/- hours. This allows you to make two days' worth of smoothies at the same time while limiting the loss of nutrients.

Sweeteners – Should you prefer to sweeten the flavor a little, the only sweetener I would recommend is Stevia. The liquid drops tend to be the easiest to regulate and get consistent flavor. Absolutely do not use any artificial sweeteners. These have been shown to be worse for you than straight sugar. Also, avoid using honey, agave, or any other traditional sweetener during the 10-Day Reset, regardless of any health claims. The reason for this is that it will negatively affect the breaking of any sugar addiction and the process of resetting your taste buds.

10-DAY PROGRAM

Eating Plan

Your daily eating plan is based on ingredients, rather than specific recipes. For each plan, I have included a shopping list of all the ingredients you will need to complete five days of the program. There is also a convenient daily checklist, so you can track and mark off each item as you consume it. This way, you are sure not to miss anything. The following Example Daily Reset Strategy gives you a daily outline of how you can successfully consume all the ingredients. That being said, there are only two rules you must follow to complete the 10-Day Bio Metabolic Reset program successfully. They are:

1. Consume all and only the ingredients listed on the daily consumption list.
2. Eat everything raw (frozen is ok, but do not cook any of the ingredients).

That is all there is to it! To make things easier, I recommend consuming the majority of your ingredients in smoothies. Not only does this make it easier to consume them, but it makes it more convenient to take with you on the go. I have included a few smoothie recipes that use all the daily ingredients as a reference, but feel free to mix things up to suit your personal tastes.

Note: *You may wish to chill your smoothie after mixing to suit your preference.*

Program Variations by Target Weight Goal

There are program variations based on different weight ranges. These variations are based on specific weight goals (not your current weight). Follow the plan and variations that are in alignment with your target weight goal.

Weekly Shopping List

This list includes 100% of the ingredients you will need for doing 5 days of your 10-Day Bio Metabolic Reset. This will help make shopping convenient and limit unnecessarily wasting food. Make sure you also get the plan specific ingredients noted in the variations following the main list. I recommend using organic ingredients whenever possible. This is especially important for the following items on your list:

- Berries
- Celery
- Spinach
- Apples

5-Day Shopping List

5-Day Shopping List			
Ingredients:	**Quantity**	**Units**	✓
Apples (fuji or gala)	2 1/2	Medium	☐
Sauerkraut (fresh)	2 1/2	Cups	☐
Watermelon (diced)	2 1/2	Cups	☐
Grapefruit	2 1/2	Medium	☐
Lemon	5	Medium	☐
Frozen Berry Mix (organic)	2 1/2	Cups	☐
Cucumber	5	Medium	☐
Celery	20	Stalks	☐
Leafy Greens (spinach or kale)	10	Cups	☐
Broccoli (chopped)	2 1/2	Cups	☐
Ginger	10	Inches	☐
Beets	1 1/4	Each	☐
Almonds, raw	1 2/3	Cups	☐
Flax seeds - Ground	15	Tablespoons	☐
Chia seeds	5	Tablespoons	☐
Coconut water	20	Ounces	☐
MCT Oil	5	Tablespoons	☐
Coconut Oil	7 1/2	Tablespoons	☐
Cinnamon - Ground	10	Teaspoons	☐
Protein Powder	5	Servings	☐
B-12 Vitamin	5	Each	☐
Liver Rescue Supplement	Max x 5	Each	☐
Colon Cleanse	Max x 5	Each	☐
Probiotic Supplement	Max x 5	Each	☐
Green Tea	5	Bags	☐
Black Tea	5-10	Bags	☐
Apple Cider Vinegar (with mother)	5	Tablespoons	☐
Water (minimum)	250	Ounces	☐

Weight Goal Program Variations

Plan A – Less than 130 pounds.

- No additional ingredients

Plan B – Between 131-165 pounds.
Additional:

- ½ cup Almonds
- 1 Apple
- 1 Grapefruit
- 60oz Water

Plan C – More than 165 pounds.
Additional:

- 1 cup Almonds
- 2 Apples
- 2 Grapefruit
- 120oz Water

Daily Consumption

Consume everything on this list plus your weight specific additional ingredients as listed on page 88 each of the 10 days of your reset.

Daily Consumption			Daily Check List				
Ingredients:	Quantity	Units	1	2	3	4	5
Apples (fuji or gala)	1/2	Medium	☐	☐	☐	☐	☐
Sauerkraut (fresh)	1/2	Cup	☐	☐	☐	☐	☐
Watermelon (diced)	1/2	Cup	☐	☐	☐	☐	☐
Grapefruit	1/2	Medium	☐	☐	☐	☐	☐
Lemon	1	Medium	☐	☐	☐	☐	☐
Frozen Berry Mix (organic)	1/2	Cup	☐	☐	☐	☐	☐
Cucumber	1	Medium	☐	☐	☐	☐	☐
Celery	4	Stalks	☐	☐	☐	☐	☐
Leafy Greens (spinach or kale)	2	Cups	☐	☐	☐	☐	☐
Broccoli (chopped)	1/2	Cup	☐	☐	☐	☐	☐
Ginger	2	Inches	☐	☐	☐	☐	☐
Beets	1/4	Each	☐	☐	☐	☐	☐
Almonds, raw	1/3	Cup	☐	☐	☐	☐	☐
Flax seeds - Ground	3	Tablespoons	☐	☐	☐	☐	☐
Chia seeds	1	Tablespoon	☐	☐	☐	☐	☐
Coconut water	4	Ounces	☐	☐	☐	☐	☐
MCT Oil	1	Tablespoon	☐	☐	☐	☐	☐
Coconut Oil	1 1/2	Tablespoons	☐	☐	☐	☐	☐
Cinnamon - Ground	2	Teaspoons	☐	☐	☐	☐	☐
Protein Powder	1	Serving	☐	☐	☐	☐	☐
Vitamin B-12	1	Each	☐	☐	☐	☐	☐
Liver Rescue Supplement	Max	Each	☐	☐	☐	☐	☐
Colon Cleanse	Max	Each	☐	☐	☐	☐	☐
Probiotic Supplement	Max	Each	☐	☐	☐	☐	☐
Green Tea	1	Bag	☐	☐	☐	☐	☐
Black Tea	1-2	Bags	☐	☐	☐	☐	☐
Apple Cider Vinegar (with mother)	1	Tablespoons	☐	☐	☐	☐	☐
Water (minimum)	50	Ounces	☐	☐	☐	☐	☐

EXAMPLE DAILY RESET STRATEGY

The following strategy and schedule tends to work well for most, but feel free to mix things up and make adjustments as needed to suit you. The important part is to consume all the ingredients listed for your Bio Metabolic Reset on each of the 10 days.

Intermittent Fast – Beginning at dark, go without food for 16 hours.

10X Fasting Tea – In the morning when you really begin to feel hungry, consume your 10X Fasting Tea to extend your fast, hopefully for the entire 16 hours.

Breaking Fast, Morning Re-Hydration – Consume the Apple Cider Detox beverage.

Meal #1 – Consume the following:

- Heavenly Bliss Smoothie

Meal #1 Supplements – Take the following supplements:

- Vitamin B-12
- Liver Rescue – 1 capsule
- Colon Cleanse – 1 capsule
- Probiotic – 1 capsule

Crunchy Snack – Celery or almonds

Meal #2 – Consume the following:

- 10X Super Smoothie
- Green Tea

Meal #2 Supplements – Take the following supplements:

- Colon Cleanse – 1 capsule

Gut Flora Builder – Eat raw sauerkraut

Crunchy Snack – Celery or almonds

Meal #3 – Consume the following:

- 10X Super Smoothie

Meal #3 Supplements – Take the following supplements:

- Liver Rescue – 1 capsule
- Colon Cleanse – 1 capsule
- Probiotic – 1 capsule

Hydration – Consume your recommended minimum of water throughout the day.

Warning

Always follow supplement manufacturer's directions and never exceed daily serving size recommendations!

RESET RECIPES

10X Super Smoothie

Put all the ingredients in a nutria-bullet (or other high-speed extracting blender). Mix for 30-60 seconds or until all ingredients are thoroughly chopped and blended.

- 1/8 - cup almonds
- 1/2 - tablespoon chia seeds
- 1-1/2 - tablespoons flaxseed (preferably pre-ground)
- 1 – inch ginger root
- 1/8 - beet
- 1/4 - cup broccoli
- 1/2 - cucumber (peeled)
- 1/4 - apple (fuji or gala – with peel, cored only)
- 2 - stocks celery
- 1/4 - grapefruit
- 1 - cup leafy greens (spinach or kale)
- 1/4 - lemon
- 12oz - cold water (adjust for desired consistency)

Heavenly Bliss Smoothie

Put all ingredients in an extractor (nutria-bullet or comparable appliance). Mix for 30-60 seconds or until all ingredients are thoroughly chopped and blended.

1/2 - cup frozen berry mix
1/2 - cup watermelon
1 - serving protein powder (plant based)
1 - teaspoon cinnamon
4oz - coconut water
4oz - cold water (adjust for desired consistency)

Apple Cider Vinegar Detox

Mix all ingredients in a mug or glass.

10oz - warm water
1 - tablespoon apple cider vinegar (raw with mother)
1 - tablespoon fresh squeezed lemon juice
Optional - add cinnamon, the more the better

10X Fasting Tea

Brew 1 or 2 bags (8-16oz) of hot tea, depending on your preference. Mix all ingredients in bullet or other high-speed mixer for 30 seconds.

8-16oz - hot water
1-2 - bags black tea
1 - tablespoon MCT oil
1-1/2 - tablespoon coconut oil

Daily Program Variations by Target Weight Goal

Consume these additional ingredients daily by adding to your smoothies or eating in addition to them.

Plan A – Less than 130 pounds.

- No variations

Plan B – Between 131-165 pounds.

- 10 Almonds
- 1/4 Apple
- 1/4 Grapefruit
- 12oz Water

Plan C – More than 165 pounds.

- 20 Almonds
- 1/2 Apple
- 1/2 Grapefruit
- 24oz Water

Q AND A

Here are answers to some of the most common questions I get asked about performing a 10-Day Bio Metabolic Reset.

Question – Is it safe?

Answer – All the items you will consume are natural and safe, unless you are allergic to any of them. That being said, there are other risks, so you should always check with your doctor before starting any health or diet program. The biggest known risk comes from health improvements to a condition that you are currently being treated for pharmaceutically. The most common is blood pressure. This program is known to lower high blood pressure; therefore, if you are taking drugs to lower it while doing this, your blood pressure may get too low. If this is you, your doctor may recommend monitoring your blood pressure more closely and possibly reducing the amount of medication you are taking to avoid this condition.

Question – Are there any side effects?

Answer – Currently, the only known side effects are weight loss and improved health.

Question – Will it be uncomfortable?

Answer – Your lifestyle and body will be going through amazing changes for the better, so you may experience some discomfort as it transitions. Any discomfort experienced will be short term and an indication that your body needed a reset. The following are some of the discomforts you may experience:

- Fatigue
- Headache
- Nausea
- Weakness

- Irritability
- Mood Swings
- Dizziness
- Hunger

Question – Is it hard to stick with it?

Answer – You can expect to have some temptations to consume some of the typical foods you are used to eating. Those moments will require a little extra willpower but should diminish as your body adapts and you see and feel the positive changes taking place.

Q AND A

Question – Is it expensive?

Answer – Ironically, doing a 10-Day reset or eating the 10X Super Health Lifestyle way is not much, if any, more expensive. In fact, if you frequently eat out, you probably spend more right now. When you eat the right high-quality foods, you do not need to eat as much. So, good food may be "more expensive", but it does not necessarily cost more to eat healthy.

Question – Is it complicated?

Answer – Actually, it could not get much simpler. The shopping list provided makes shopping efficient and simple. The foods you will eat are the same every day, so you can prepare in advance the ingredients for multiple meals/smoothies at the same time. Then it should only take you a few minutes to prepare each meal.

Question – Is it time consuming?

Answer – If you currently cook your meals at home, it should take you the same or less time to prepare your reset foods. If you eat out or do a combination, it is still not likely to take any more time than what you would currently spend obtaining and preparing food. If you consume your reset foods as smoothies, they can be taken on the go, making eating even more efficient and saving time.

Question – Do I have to know how to cook?

Answer – Absolutely not, all the ingredients are eaten raw. You will need to measure, cut, prep, and blend some of the ingredients, but the recipes are easy to follow, so anyone can do it.

LIFE AFTER RESET

A Lifestyle for Life

10X SUPER HEALTH LIFESTYLE

If you want to maintain a superior level of health after completing your 10-Day Bio Metabolic Reset, this is your next step. Now that you have retaken control of your health, it is time to develop a new lifestyle that will easily support and maintain it. Good health does not need to be cumbersome, nor do you need to buy all kinds of special foods or supplements to achieve it. The 10X Super Health Lifestyle is based on readily available foods and does not require excessive exercise. The following section will give you a general guideline that, if followed, can help you easily maintain your ideal body weight and an optimum level of health. Great health starts with nutritional balance.

80/20 NUTRITIONAL BALANCE

The primary balance involves getting 80% of your calories from plant-based whole foods and 20% from high value animal-based.

80% Plant-Based Whole Foods

Vegetables & Fruits	Nuts & Seeds	Legumes	Whole Grains
40%	20%	10%	10%

20% Animal-Based

High Value Animal-Based
20%

Although this is a general guideline, it is actually the goal. By general, I mean there is no need to stress if you are not spot on. Focus your primary eating on the larger categories and keep your balance in mind when making food decisions. Eating should be enjoyable and not cause stress. The goal is to work you into a lifetime of good eating habits, so give yourself some time to transition while you get your balance and routine in place.

Balanced Calorie Method

Once you reach your ideal weight and health status, you will surely want to maintain it. Eating the right foods is an important part of the health equation, but you will also want to have a good point of reference for how much of each food category you should be consuming. This will be calculated based on your personalized maintenance caloric intake and specific details, like age, gender, height, weight, and activity level.

So, what does 20% of your diet being nuts and seeds look like? I know that might be a bit confusing, so here is a simple method for maintaining a healthy balance. Although I am not big on counting calories, they can be a useful resource for understanding your ideal nutritional balance. Use the following Food Calorie Balance calculator to convert the Nutritional Balance percentages into your own personalized Food Calorie Balance.

Here is an example calorie breakdown based on the typical 2000 calorie diet used for most nutritional calculations.

Example Total Calories 2000

Vegetable and Fruits

Total calories *2000* x .40 = *800*

Nuts & Seeds

Total calories *2000* x .20 = *400*

Legumes

Total calories *2000* x .10 = *200*

Whole Grains

Total calories *2000* x .10 = *200*

High Value Animal Based

Total calories *2000* x .20 = *400*

Example Food Calorie Balance

80% Plant-Based Whole Foods

Vegetables & Fruits	Nuts & Seeds	Legumes	Whole Grains
800	**400**	**200**	**200**

20% Animal-Based

High Value Animal-Based
400

Your Food Calorie Balance

Work through the following steps to create your personalized Food Calorie Balance. If you do not know what your daily maintenance caloric intake is, use the free calculator at the following website to find out:

http://www.calculator.net/calorie-calculator.html

Use your ideal weight when performing the calculation. Then, enter your personalized information and complete each of the formulas.

Total Calories _____

Vegetable and Fruits

Total calories _____ x .40 = _____

Nuts & Seeds

Total calories _____ x .20 = _____

Legumes

Total calories _____ x .10 = _____

Whole Grains

Total calories _____ x .10 = _____

High Value Animal Based

Total calories _____ x .20 = _____

Personalized Food Balance

80% Plant-Based Whole Foods

Vegetables & Fruits	Nuts & Seeds	Legumes	Whole Grains

20% Animal-Based

High Value Animal-Based

Our bodies are adaptable, so food is not an exact science. If you are within a reasonable proximity of balance, your diet will be supportive of good health. Our bodies were actually designed to deal with things like food scarcity and variations in the types of nutrients consumed. So, if your calories fluctuate or you eat a little more or less of certain categories some days over others, your body will adapt. That being said, there are two areas of the typical Western Diet that you want to be sure to avoid.

Over Consuming Harmful Foods

Your body will have a hard time maintaining good health if you are consuming an overabundance of chemical laden, processed, and modified foods. Some of which are things like commercially farmed foods, sugar laden drinks, highly refined grains (like flour), refined oils, and large quantities of added sugar or salt. These are overused and prevalent in most of the manufactured and pre-packaged foods available these days. Since our bodies were never designed or prepared to process these types of products, eating them can be harmful, especially over a long period of time.

Obviously, it is unreasonable to expect you will not consume any commercially farmed, processed, or modified foods, but there are some things you can do to reduce your overall level of exposure to harmful foods. Things like doing some research to choose companies that are the least offensive, as well as eating organic varieties when possible, are a great start. Also, try to prepare more of your meals from individual ingredients and whole foods, not pre-packed kits.

Long-Term Nutrient Deficiencies

If you have a shortage of certain nutrients for short periods of time, although not ideal, your body can adapt in some pretty amazing ways. Then, as long as you replenish these regularly, your body will rebalance and restore its reserves. Eating quality foods based on the 10X Super Health Lifestyle nutritional balance will help you avoid any long-term deficiencies.

10X SUPER HEALTH FOOD PRINCIPLES

Once you know your food balance, then you will want to focus on these principles that will help you navigate the maze of deceptive food marketing. Using these basic principles will help you avoid getting lost in the marketing and food hype that is so prevalent these days. Here are some general rules to follow for each food category.

Vegetables & Fruits (40%)

You want to obtain 40% of your calories from vegetables and fruits, with an emphasis on vegetables. This includes tubers (most people would automatically recognize these as vegetables like carrots and yams). The larger assortment of colors, the better, and minimize the high starch vegetables like potatoes. Although still vegetables, these will have high calorie and high carb to low beneficial nutrient ratios.

Remember, our bodies can adapt to short-term deficiencies in nutrients but ultimately needs a good diversity. The best strategy when it comes to vegetables and fruits is to eat a broad spectrum of many types. So try to mix it up and eat a good assortment. Here are a few more tips for making the best choices.

Colorful – Eat a great diversity of colors, the deeper and richer the color, typically the more nutritious.

Limit Starch – Limit high carb starchy vegetables, like potatoes, these are the least beneficial.

Watch Sugar – Do not replace a sugar addiction with overconsuming fruits that have a naturally high sugar content.

Do Not Juice Fruits – This may sound contrary to all the juicing hype these days, but all juice is not created equal or even beneficial for you. This is especially the case when it comes to juicing oranges, apples, and other sweet fruits. Drinking these fruits with the fiber removed essentially turns them into soda, some containing even higher quantities of sugar. This high sugar content with no fiber, turns otherwise healthy fruits into a blood glucose spiking beverage.

Nuts and Seeds (20%)

Your nuts and seeds will help you maintain a good level of protein and healthy fats in your diet. They are also an important source of disease preventing nutrients and fiber.

Just like vegetables and fruits, there are many types of nuts and seeds. The most beneficial approach is to eat a diverse array of them. Each nut and seed will have its own strong points and good benefits, but trying to single out which ones you should eat to obtain a certain attribute is lots of work and unnecessary. Nuts are great for snacking, and seeds can be great additions to smoothies. Here is a list of some nuts and seeds I recommend making a priority.

Great Nuts and Seeds

Nuts

- Almonds
- Pecans
- Walnuts
- Brazil Nuts
- Pistachios
- Cashews

Seeds

- Flaxseed (ground)
- Chia
- Hemp
- Sesame
- Pumpkin
- Sunflower

Peanuts are not Nuts!

Sad but true, peanuts are actually legumes and do not share the same health benefits of most nuts. That is not to say they are all bad. They are just not nuts and should be judged and consumed for what they are.

Legumes (10%)

Legumes will help promote regularity, provide you with protein and other heart healthy nutrients, and help make you feel satiated. As with anything that has scientific benefits, sometimes there are also opposing negative attributes present, and legumes have some. That being said, if you avoided everything that has a bad attribute, you would likely starve or die from lack of something in one of those evil ingredients. So do not avoid legumes; just consume them in moderation and prioritize the best ones.

The Good

For a plant-based food, legumes are high in protein, contain a good amount of fiber, as well as other great nutrients.

The Bad

Anti-Nutrients – Legumes are known for containing anti-nutrients, which essentially can interfere with the body's ability to absorb certain nutrients.

Lectins and Saponins – Legumes contain lectins and saponins, which are resistant to digestion and have been known to affect the cells lining the intestinal tract, which can lead to a condition know as "leaky gut".

Phytic Acid – This is found in all plants and can impair the absorption of some minerals.

It is Not All Bad

All those things sound scary, but many are offset and compensated for by other things you will be eating. Unless you have a current case of "leaky gut" or other medical condition that warrants the elimination of legumes from your diet, the benefits likely outweigh the bad. When making selections, lean towards lower starch legumes, like peas and lentils.

Whole Grains (10%)

Whole grains will provide a good source of dietary fiber, as well as minerals and other nutrients. Grains are typically an inexpensive source of nutrients (the good part) and are therefore typically overconsumed (the bad part). Due to its low cost and easy production, it is also a food that has been highly modified and is overused in processed and packaged foods.

It is extremely important that you actually consume "Whole Grains." Many food manufacturers label products "made with whole grains," but it may actually be blended with highly refined grains, which have substantial negative health effects. There are also grains known for being much better for you. Use the following information to help guide your grain choices.

Grain Choices

Always shoot for whole grains. Highly refined flours are not great but are better when of the whole grain variety. Whole grain means it contains all the parts of the original grain. A good rule of thumb, the least refined variety of any food is typically the healthiest.

Preferred	Moderation	Avoid
• Quinoa	• Oats (steel	• Highly
• Buckwheat	cut)	Refined
• Millet	• Whole Wheat	• Highly
• Amaranth	• Rye	Processed
• Brown Rice	• Corn (Non-	• White Rice
• Black Rice	GMO)	• White Flour
• Wild Rice	• Pre-packaged	• GMOs

Obviously, if you are allergic to anything, you should avoid it. There has been an increase in celiac disease recently, and whether due to highly refined gluten containing grains or gluten grains in general, this may be a sign that consuming gluten containing products may not be a good idea.

High Value Animal Based (20%)

High Value Animal based foods are included in the 10X Super Health Lifestyle eating plan due to their beneficial effects on gut bacteria, obtaining Omega-3 fatty acids, and being a natural source of vitamin B12. If you are vegan or just do not want to eat animal products, you can eliminate this category if you like. Just be sure, if you go primarily or 100% plant based, to consume enough of the right sources or use supplements to avoid any deficiencies in these areas.

I know many will miss having that big slab of steak, but a better way to think of and use meats in your diet is as a flavoring ingredient, not the main course.

The way most animal products are produced today warrant severely minimizing or eliminating their consumption. I am speaking in regard to health here. The humane aspect of it is also appalling, but that is more of a moral judgment than a health related one. Regardless of which side of that you come down on, here are some major considerations to help steer your decisions.

Meat – Should always be free range and organic. Animals should be raised consuming their natural diets, i.e., grass for cows. Any meat should be in whole form, no ground products (you have no idea what is in there, and they do not tend to grind the best meats; often it is primarily the leftover offcuts). Any red meat should be extra lean. Chicken and other meats are often plumped (injected with salt water or other solutions). You do not want this for two reasons:

1. You are partially paying for water or an unknown solution by the pound, not meat.
2. There is unnecessary added salt, deceiving you of the true flavor of the product.

Eggs – Should be organic from chickens that are free-range, cage free, or pastured.

Seafood – Should be wild caught, and although canned is acceptable, fresh is always preferred. There are numerous varieties of seafood, but for a quick reference to help you choose the good and avoid the bad, here are some general recommendations:

Preferred	Moderation	Avoid
• Anchovies	• Albacore Tuna	• Farmed
• Clams		• Bluefin Tuna
• Oysters	• Sablefish	• Shark
• Sardines	• Salmon	• Swordfish
• Scallops		• Tilapia

There is certainly other seafood out there, and if there is something specific you like, I would recommend doing a little research, so you know what you are eating. Check into the toxic chemical levels it is known to contain, as well as whether it is threatened due to overfishing.

Dairy Products – These should be severely limited or totally eliminated. Frankly, I believe there is more harm than benefit to most dairy products. Milk should be avoided 100%. This is a guaranteed way to get high doses of things you do not want, like casein. If you need scientific proof you do not want to consume casein, just do a little Google research.

Sure, milk and other dairy products have been touted for building strong bones and being good sources of nutrients we need, but unfortunately, it comes in a package combined with things we do not. Everything milk and dairy has that we need can be adequately obtained from better, non-harmful sources. Dairy is also a major allergen, which should be an indicator we do not want or need it. Also consider this; we are the only species that drinks milk after the initial stages of life.

If you do consume dairy, make sure it is from the highest quality sources, like grass fed animals, organic and skip the low fat/no fat versions.

Goat and Sheep Milk – When available, it is preferable for most dairy products like cheese and yogurt. Goat and sheep milk do not contain A1 Casein, which can be inflammatory and cause digestion issues for many people.

Dairy Substitutes – Like most things, when you try to replicate something bad, you eliminate some bad elements while adding others. This is very true in dairy alternatives. I am not saying they are all bad, because they are not, but you have to research them carefully to know for sure. Some are made with things like vegetable oils, which you should not consume anymore than dairy. Regardless of the health quality of the substitute, the price will definitely be higher, which may make a substitute cost prohibitive.

If you do have an allergy to dairy, obviously, you should eliminate it. For the rest of us, severely limiting the amount we consume may be good enough to maintain a reasonably high level of health. By severely limit, I mean, if you want pizza, put about 20% of the cheese that would normally be found on one. Do not have cheese or other dairy with every meal or even every day. Use it as an occasional flavor enhancer, not a primary ingredient.

Hormone and Antibiotic Free – Things like milk, farmed fish, and poorly raised/produced meats come loaded with all kinds of hormones and antibiotics you do not want in your diet. Indicators like organic, hormone, and antibiotic free can help direct your choices, so do your homework to limit your exposure to these harmful substances.

HEALTHY EATING THAT TASTE GREAT

Spices and Seasoning

Herbs and most spices have a health range from neutral to highly beneficial. The primary flavoring components you want to avoid are the "Bad Three" which are typically overused in processed foods: unhealthy fats, salt, and sugar. Peppers (recommend fresh ground), especially of the spicy variety, are great for high flavor impact (if you can handle it). Almost all herbs and spices not included in the "bad three" are fair game and can be used liberally. Most commercially available liquid seasonings and dressings will be loaded with sugar and crap you do not want, so try to avoid or screen these carefully. Mustard is typically great, but ketchup tends to be loaded with sugar and other bad ingredients.

Seasoning List

If you have not done a lot of home cooking, spices can be confusing and expensive. To help give a little guidance, I have created a list of 21 seasonings that I believe to be healthy, versatile, and a must for every kitchen.

21 Must Have Seasonings

- Allspice
- Basil
- Bay Leaves
- Black Peppercorns
- Cayenne Pepper
- Chili Powder
- Cinnamon Powder
- Curry Powder
- Garlic Powder
- Ginger Root Powder
- Ground Cumin
- Himalayan or Sea Salt
- Nutmeg
- Onion Powder
- Oregano
- Red Pepper Flakes
- Rosemary
- Sage
- Smoked Paprika
- Thyme
- Turmeric

Some other seasonings you may want to have on hand in fresh form are garlic, parsley, cilantro, and ginger. Around my house, fresh garlic, red pepper flakes, and black pepper are the most commonly used flavor enhancers.

Oils/Fats

There are many great oils that can serve different purposes. For high temperature cooking or frying, you need to be a little more selective due to some healthier oils having low smoke points, which can make them toxic when overheated. For frying, if you are into that type of food, our recommendation is coconut oil, which has been shown to be stable for long periods of time at temperatures up to 365 degrees. For consumption as an added ingredient or for flavoring, I recommend primarily olive oil (extra virgin cold pressed), although there are some other good alternatives. Here is a short list of common good and bad oils:

Preferred	Avoid
Extra Virgin Olive Oil (cold pressed)	Canola Oil
Almond Oil	Vegetable Oil
Avocado Oil	Safflower Oil
Flax Oil	Soybean Oil
Hemp Oil	Sunflower Oil
Sesame Seed Oil	Corn Oil
Walnut Oil	Palm Oil
Butter (limited use)	Peanut Oil
Ghee (limited use)	Shortening
	Alternative Spreads

If you are in a transitional phase of the program (doing it as a means of weight loss or improved health), I advise strictly sticking to the plant-based oils. If you are not and wish to use other products for baking or other purposes, I would recommend butter or ghee from grass fed animals. Hopefully, any use of these would be kept to a minimum as they are dairy products, but I feel they are the lesser of the evils.

There may be some reasonable alternatives in the form of mixed product spreads, but this is an area of great deception when it comes to health benefits and consequences. Most will contain vegetable oils, water, and other ingredients that skew the bad ingredients but really do not make the product any healthier than butter. Due to those facts, avoid spreads unless you are a scientist that understands what they are and can verify their health affects.

Note: *Avoid vegetable oils. There are many vegetable oils and different types of oils marketed as healthier alternatives. Many contain GMO's or are just not healthy due to the way they are processed. This is why, when it comes to oils and fats, I included a list of ingredients to use. By following the included guideline, you can avoid the potential confusion and know you are eating ingredients of the healthier type.*

FOOD QUALITY

All food is not equal, not even close, especially not these days. With genetic engineering, an abundance of chemicals used during production, scientific modification, and re-blending to lower the cost in packaged foods, it is hard to know what you are actually getting. Far more important than counting calories when it comes to your health is the quality of your food. Major manufacturers go out of their way with labeling and marketing to make you feel like you are making a healthy and wise choice, when in reality, you are oftentimes buying crap food-like products in disguise.

I believe the organic, free range, grass fed, buy local and most of the other healthy food mantras support better quality ingredients. If you can afford it, I would recommend going that direction. That being said, I knew, when I put this program together, it had to work for everyone, regardless of financial situation or philosophical view. Here are a few food rules that will allow you to make much better food buying decisions.

Always Look at the Ingredients – Never assume by the label you know what is inside. If it has a nutrition label, check the ingredients. If you do not know what an ingredient is, put it back. There are almost always going to be some preservatives in a shelf product. I will not say 100% are bad, but when the list of unknown ingredients grows, it is likely a chemical cocktail that you should not be consuming. Processed and pre-packaged foods are oftentimes filled with hidden, unhealthy, and addictive ingredients. There are 50+/- names for sugars and artificial sweeteners. Do you know them? I do not, and I do not want to have to know them. Quality food manufacturers will limit the use of harmful ingredients in their products; therefore, the ingredients list will be on the shorter side and all things you will likely recognize (food).

As you start reading labels, you will find there are a lot of foods out there that you thought were healthy that, in reality, you should not be eating. This may be disappointing, but it clearly indicates one source of our obesity and chronic disease epidemics. You will also see how almost anyone can get confused and make poor health choices, even if they are trying hard not to do so.

Organics Versus Conventional

Obviously, organics would always be preferred. That being said, there are some specific ingredients that rank of higher importance when it comes to buying organic. This is due to the way they retain pesticides, may be GMO, or likely contain other bad elements from the industrialized food production process. This is not a complete list or meant to be a promotion of the items on the "either way" list. Use this guide to help you focus on where spending more money will get you the most health benefit for the buck.

Organic or Conventional?

Organic

- Animal Products
- Legumes & Grains
- Nuts and Seeds
- Apples
- Berries (all kinds)
- Celery
- Leafy Greens
- Broccoli
- Tofu

Either Way

- Oranges
- Grapefruits
- Bananas
- Carrots
- Fruits/Vegetables (when eaten after skin removal)

THINGS TO AVOID

Highly Refined Grains – Eat only whole grains. Many flours are often highly refined and have parts of the grains removed to make them more desirable. This gives them the same effect as sugar, once inside your body. Your body quickly turns refined carbohydrates into blood glucose (a simple sugar), once you consume it. When you eat whole grains, the fiber is still present, which slows down your body's ability to turn it into sugar (that is a good thing), thereby reducing the blood sugar spike and need for insulin.

Since sugar was not found in abundance in nature, your body was designed to turn many different types of foods into the sugar it needs. Food manufacturers have discovered that sugar has addictive qualities. Some studies have shown it to be even more addictive than cocaine. That is why most food manufacturers use it in abundance and put it in virtually every food they sell. Hence, we have an exploding epidemic of obesity, Type 2 diabetes, and other avoidable chronic illnesses.

To help protect your health, you will want to be sure that any grain-based products you consume are made with whole grains. This can get a little confusing, since oftentimes, things are marketed as "made with whole grains" but also include highly refined grains. A simple reading of the ingredients label will tell you all you need to know.

No Added Sugar – When you find added sugar, this is a telltale sign that a manufacturer is trying to play and profit on the average person's addiction to sugar. Sure, if you are buying a cake, it is going to have added sugar. It is a desert and to be expected (cake by the way is not on the plan). What I am talking about is added sugar in things like fruits, oatmeal, tomato sauce, ketchup etc., places it should not be.

To clarify, things like apples have naturally occurring sugar, so if the ingredients include apples, you may have a higher sugar content without any added sugar. This is why the ingredients list is the most important part of the nutrition label. 5 grams of sugar in a package of applesauce may be ok, unless the ingredients list includes apples and sugar or artificial sweeteners. These items should be avoided, and any other products made by that brand should be subject to higher scrutiny.

Minimal or No Processed/Packaged Foods – It is understandable that people look to packaged/processed foods to help expedite the cooking process. We live in hectic times. Unfortunately, packaging food allows manufacturers to do some pretty unscrupulous things to your food. Many of these things reduce the nutritional value and oftentimes make the food detrimental to your health and weight management goals.

I promote finding simple recipes you like that you can easily cook with ingredients from the perimeter of the supermarket. Almost all the unhealthy fat generators are in the center of the store. If you typically eat from that area, you will likely never be able to control your weight or maintain good health. Almost all foods that are not in their whole form (as they would be in nature) have been processed and modified for profits and possibly even addictive qualities. It is hard, if not impossible, to lose or maintain your weight when you have a longing for another hit of your favorite addiction.

Minimal Added Salt – If you are eating any packaged foods, you are probably getting an abundance of salt, likely more than you need. Once again, salt is a substance our bodies need that had not previously been so readily available; therefore, we naturally crave it. Companies take advantage of this natural craving and use salt excessively to keep us coming back for more.

When you eat the 10X Super Health Lifestyle and prepare the majority of your own foods, you will probably want to add salt. In this case, adding some salt is ok, since you will not already be consuming an overabundance. When you do add salt, do not add it in excessive amounts, negating your health gains. Never use traditional table salt. Stick to sea, pink Himalayan, or Kosher salt.

GMOs

Genetically modified organisms (GMOs) are essentially foods that have been reengineered for faster growth, rot and bug resistance, or other desirable attributes. All those things sound great, but there is a lot of controversy about what this means regarding its nutritional value and more specifically the value for human consumption. Many of these GMO products are refined and turned into biofuels or used as animal feed, but more and more are reaching grocery store shelves.

Consuming GMOs is a personal choice we must all make. As for me, I avoid GMOs to the greatest extent possible. I am not saying they are good or bad, but when man starts playing god, I will take a long-term wait and see approach. The current reality is that food related chronic illnesses, like diabetes, high cholesterol, high blood pressure, heart disease etc., have skyrocketed in recent years. Are GMOs the cause? Is it the refining process? The chemical additives? The high consumption of low nutrient obesity causing foods? Eating GMO foods is a decision we must each make for ourselves. If you want to avoid all those negative food attributes and skip being part of the experiment, go GMO free.

I value avoiding GMOs more than I value an organic only approach. I am in no way saying that is the right choice, just my opinion and decision. We do not know with any certainty what eating genetically modified food will do to our genes or health over the long term, so I recommend opting out.

CONCLUSION

Hopefully, all this information has provided a little more clarity in how you can obtain the highest level of health, while more easily maintaining a healthy body weight. If you feel a little overwhelmed and lost, that is understandable. Keep it simple and start by focusing on mastering a few key elements like these:

- Severely limit processed and packaged foods
- Eliminate added sugars
- Greatly reduce or eliminate your dairy intake
- Do not drink sugar beverages (sports drinks, soda, or even fruit juices)
- Increase your consumption of plant based foods, especially colorful vegetables

Get Support

Reach out to family or friends to help you get on and stay on the path to good health, this will greatly increase your chances of being successful and sticking with it. Support has been shown to be one of the strongest contributors to succeeding at any major life change, especially a diet. If you do not have good options for support from family or friends, consider joining a related Facebook group or other outside resource.

A Simple Request

Thanks for reading this book. I hope you have enjoyed it.

If you have, I have one simple request to ask. Could you please leave an honest review for it on Amazon.com?

This will only take you a minute but will make a huge difference in our ability to get this message out and help other people improve their health situation.

In a world dominated by large corporate interest, our voice is small, so every review counts and helps make it a little louder.

Best wishes and live healthy!
Dan

TRACKING YOUR RESULTS

RESULTS LOG

Use this form to track your weight daily and blood pressure weekly. Check your weight every morning after using the restroom and before consuming anything. Do not drink alcohol or highly caffeinated drinks before testing blood pressure.

Beginning Blood Pressure

Systolic:	Diastolic:	Pulse:
_____	_____	_____

Daily Weight Log

Day 1 Weight: _____	Day 6 Weight: _____
Day 2 Weight: _____	Day 7 Weight: _____
Day 3 Weight: _____	Day 8 Weight: _____
Day 4 Weight: _____	Day 9 Weight: _____
Day 5 Weight: _____	Day 10 Weight: _____

Ending Blood Pressure

Systolic:	Diastolic:	Pulse:
_____	_____	_____

CAPTURE THE JOURNEY

Throughout your 10-Day Bio Metabolic Reset, one of your psychological strength building exercises will be to keep a daily journal. Journaling has many beneficial aspects. One of the most beneficial is the increased ability to clarify your thoughts and feelings. Better understanding the changes you will be going through can help give you the strength to press on when you are feeling challenged. Feel free to do this at any time of the day that works for you, although doing it at the same set time each day tends to work best.

Day 1 Journal

Date: _____ **How are you feeling?** ☐☐☐☐☐☐☐☐☐

Worse – Same - Better

Congratulations, your first day has been completed! Document your feelings, struggles, pains, accomplishments, successes etc. How hard was the day? Are you taking it in stride or battling some opposing demons?

_____

_____

_____

_____

_____

_____

_____

_____

_____

_____

_____

_____

140

Day 2 Journal

Date: _____ **How are you feeling?** ☐☐☐☐☐☐☐☐☐☐

Worse – Same - Better

Yahoo, another day completed! You are already 20% of the way through the program and approaching the most challenging days. Document your current thoughts and feelings. If you are struggling, is there anything you feel you need to do to be sure you stick with the program?

_____

_____

_____

_____

_____

_____

_____

_____

_____

_____

_____

_____

_____

_____

Day 3 Journal

Date: _____ **How are you feeling?** ☐☐☐☐☐☐☐☐☐☐

Worse – Same - Better

Day 3, this is known for being one of the hardest. You may want to focus on staying busy to help keep you distracted from food and any hunger pangs. Are you staying out of environments that might lead you to cheat? If not, now would be a good time to formulate a plan for doing so.

_____

_____

_____

_____

_____

_____

_____

_____

_____

_____

_____

_____

_____

142

Day 4 Journal

Date: _____ **How are you feeling?** ☐☐☐☐☐☐☐☐☐☐
Worse – Same - Better

You are doing great and almost halfway there. Have you been sticking to the program 100%? What changes have you noticed so far? Has this been challenging, or are you taking it in stride? A couple more days and the worst will be over, then things should get easier.

_____

_____

_____

_____

_____

_____

_____

_____

_____

_____

_____

_____

_____

Day 5 Journal

Date: _____ **How are you feeling?** ☐☐☐☐☐☐☐☐☐☐

Worse – Same - Better

This is hump day; you are halfway done. If you have gotten this far, I know you are the type that will stick with it until the end. This might be a good time to start thinking about what changes you will make and how your diet will look after your reset. What is the next step in your health transition? How will you maintain these gains?

_____

_____

_____

_____

_____

_____

_____

_____

_____

_____

_____

_____

_____

Day 6 Journal

Date: _____ **How are you feeling?** ☐☐☐☐☐☐☐☐☐☐

Worse – Same - Better

Hopefully, by now, you have settled into an efficient routine and gotten beyond any of the initial discomforts. Have the smoothie tastes grown on you? Could you see incorporating a daily 10X Super Smoothie into your future diet? How are you feeling about your progress?

_____

_____

_____

_____

_____

_____

_____

_____

_____

_____

_____

_____

_____

Day 7 Journal

Date: _____ **How are you feeling?** ☐☐☐☐☐☐☐☐☐☐
Worse – Same - Better

Only a couple days left. Internally, your body has already undergone some major health changes, and the detoxification process is in full force. Are you staying up on your additional water intake? Your body needs to purge a lot of toxins during this process, so this additional fluid will help aid in flushing your system.

_____

_____

_____

_____

_____

_____

_____

_____

_____

_____

_____

_____

_____

Day 8 Journal

Date: _____ **How are you feeling?** □□□□□□□□□□

Worse – Same - Better

Will you adjust your future diet to incorporate the principles of a 10X Super Health Lifestyle or some other dietary lifestyle for maintaining good health? Have or will you make some long-term physical activity level changes in your lifestyle that will support good health?

_____

_____

_____

_____

_____

_____

_____

_____

_____

_____

_____

_____

_____

Day 9 Journal

Date: _____ **How are you feeling?**   ☐☐☐☐☐☐☐☐☐☐
Worse – Same - Better

Almost finished! Have you tried some of the other strategies for improving your health? Things like making sure you get enough sleep, eating based on your circadian rhythm, and stress reduction. Did you give up coffee, alcohol, or something else you enjoy while doing this program? What are your plans for these once finished?

_____

_____

_____

_____

_____

_____

_____

_____

_____

_____

_____

_____

Day 10 Journal

Date: _____ **How are you feeling?** ☐☐☐☐☐☐☐☐☐☐

Worse – Same - Better

Congratulations! You did it! The 10-Day Bio Metabolic Reset is one of the most aggressive life-changing programs out there, so this is a big accomplishment. Is there someone else you think might benefit from this program? Will you tell them about it and share your results? Should you move on to the 10X Super Health Lifestyle program, rest assured, after completing this, you will easily be able to do it. No matter what you choose to do, I hope you will make your health a priority and incorporate some lifelong habits that will make it a reality.

_____

_____

_____

_____

_____

_____

_____

_____

Celebration Time, You're Finished!

About The Author

Before I began the 10X Super Health Lifestyle, I was overweight with stage one hypertension. In just over 45 days after doing an aggressive reset, followed by some 10X Super Health Lifestyle burn and detox sessions, I hit my target weight, and my blood pressure was perfect. Following these great results, I adopted the 10X Super Health food principles and maintain an 80% plant-based whole foods and 20% high value animal products diet. This has made maintaining my weight, blood pressure, and overall health extremely easy. Since adopting this lifestyle, my weight has never varied by over 5 pounds, and I rarely have to think about calories or how much I am eating.

Shortly after completing my initial weight loss and health transformation, my mom was diagnosed as pre-diabetic. I knew the 10X principles help prevent diabetes. After doing extensive additional research, I asked her to try this program and see if it would help reverse her diabetes. She did, and at her next visit to her doctor (the one where they were going to look to start prescribing her drugs to treat it), she was diagnosed as healthy and out of the diabetic range. She has since continued to live the 10X Super Health Lifestyle, and her doctors remain impressed by her weight loss and improved overall health.

I knew this program offered easy weight loss and substantial health benefits, so I shared it with my brother. He was 100 plus pounds overweight and on numerous medications. He decided to give it a shot, and the weight rapidly began to drop off (he has already lost over 80 pounds). He has also eliminated all but one of his medications. Today, he is much healthier, has more energy, and lives a far more active lifestyle.

Since seeing these major life-changing health improvements firsthand, I have made sharing the 10X Super Health Lifestyle my mission. I hope you too will join us and live a 10X Super Health Lifestyle.

www.10xsuperhealth.com

Made in the USA
Columbia, SC
27 September 2020